IF THE SAVIOR IS NOT SAFE
HOW CAN HE SAVE?
The challenges facing physicians today

Alaa Abd-Elsayed, MD, MPH

The information provided in this book is based on best knowledge and currently available literature.

First edition, 2019.
ISBN: 9781078379939

Other books published by the author:
Chronic pain: the patient and family journey
Pain: a review guide
Infusion therapy for pain, headache and related condition

Dedication

To my parents, my wife and my two beautiful kids
Maro and George

Table of contents

Preface

The medical profession has undergone significant changes over the past few decades. Stories about major issues facing physicians such as burnout, leaving the medical profession, and physician suicide are becoming increasingly common.

A shortage of physicians currently existents in the USA and in several countries worldwide. This shortage is increasing to a point that it is currently impacting patient care in some areas and will likely only worsen in the coming years unless significant changes are made to the current culture of healthcare.

I have witnessed many changes in the health system during my career and have watched some colleagues who suffered so much and ended up committing suicide or quitting medicine. I started searching literature for statistics and numbers to confirm my observations, and the results were even more surprising and shocking than I expected.

There are significant issues that physicians are encountering that will lead to a huge shortage in the next decade. Patients simply will not have providers in certain areas to treat them, the wait time will be longer, access will be difficult, physicians will experience more burn out and the situation will continue to deteriorate.

I hope there will be efforts to address the issues physicians encounter to make sure we have enough HAPPY physicians who can provide the best care to our patients.

I hope this book will be a resource for potential applicants to medical schools, current medical students, patients, other health care support providers, politicians and the public to make sure they understand the medical culture and the challenges physicians encounter. Only when the current challenges are understood can real change occur.

I see the issues from both sides. I am a physician who deals with career challenges, but I am also a patient and a family member who wants a physician who will provide me and my family with the best care possible.

The USA has one of the greatest health care systems in the world, but the savior is not safe anymore. The savior needs to be safe so we all can be saved.

Alaa Abd-Elsayed, MD, MPH

OVERVIEW OF MEDICAL TRAINING

Physicians go through extensive study and training to attain their medical degree. After completing 4 years of an undergraduate program, physician candidates continue onto four years of medical school. Following medical school, residency is another 4 to 7 years or more of training. In addition, many physicians choose to complete advanced fellowship training which spans at least another 1 to 3 years.

Medical school includes many extremely rigorous classes and exams. Unlike other professional schools, if a medical student fails any exam or scores poorly, this will be reported in the Dean's letter when they apply for residency. As such, the study of medicine itself carries a huge risk with no room for failure. In addition, there are three United States Medical Licensing exams that a student will have to take. A student cannot repeat an exam if they pass with a low score, but a low score may cause them to seriously struggle, possibly interfering with their ability to complete their studies and pursue a career in medicine.

That's why medical students stress out about classes and exams during their medical school, knowing that any failure will count against them and may jeopardize their career all together.

Medical school requires several hours of studying daily and the days are typically long and exhausting, full of competing demands between caring for patients, attending lectures, preparing journal clubs, scholarly activities, studying, reading literature, preparing for exams, and more. And most importantly, the trainee must prioritize keeping everyone happy.

Assuming the medical student completes medical school without problems, they will apply for residency to specialize in a certain field in medicine such as orthopedic surgery, anesthesiology, or dermatology, amongst others. Some specialties are definitely more competitive than others and a student has to excel in their medical school studies to be able to get to the top specialties which eventually offer more income and better life opportunities.

During the 5-month application and interview process students apply online for the programs they are interested in, wait for interview invites, and then travel for interviews. At the end of the interview season, the students rank the programs based on their preference, and programs also rank the students.

When a student and a program both select each other, a "match" occurs. The match results are distributed in March, where the student will find out which of their top-ranked residency programs also chose them. In some cases, students do not match, and need to quickly apply for programs that still have openings, even if it is not their desired field of study.

Even upon admittance to their residency, aspiring physicians will soon recognize, this is just the beginning of a long road. From this point, the duration of training varies from specialty to specialty. For example, internal medicine takes 3 years, 4 years for anesthesiology, and up to 7 years for general surgery and neurosurgery.

Typically, three years is the least number of years a resident will spend in training. During residency, the residents will mostly receive an evaluation on a daily basis from their designated supervisors. In addition, some programs include evaluations from additional personnel, e.g. nurses and other employees of the hospital. Thus, a resident will have to excel every day in all aspects to receive good evaluations. Bad evaluations, especially if recurrent, can lead to various consequences, and can impact future opportunities.

During the residency training, there will be an annual training exam. This exam is made as a practice for the final board exam after finishing the residency training. Again, if a resident score lower than the allowed percentile by their program, there might be consequences.

After finishing residency, many residents will elect to complete further training, otherwise known as a fellowship. A fellowship allows the resident to subspecialize in a particular field. For example, I finished my Anesthesiology training in 4 years and then performed 1 year of fellowship training in Pain Medicine. Each specialty will have different fellowship opportunities, and the fellowship typically spans from 1 to 3 years, with some extending beyond this time period. If a trainee decides to specialize in the care of children, even more years of training are required.

During the fellowship training, the fellow will receive evaluations from all their supervisors and personnel they work with. Also, they will have a training exam during fellowship to prepare them for the subspecialty board. In addition, as during residency, if the fellow does not receive good

5

evaluations or scores low in the in-training exam, there might be consequences of different degrees.

During this whole time, starting with medical school and ending with fellowship, trainees are simply walking on "egg shells." There is no room for error not only medically, but also in other skills as communication, professionalism, patient experience, and more.

MEDICAL SCHOOL

Medical students face a variety of challenges. A recent research study published by the Journal of the American Medical Association indicated that 27% of medical students were diagnosed with depression or presented with associated symptoms. In addition, 11% reported suicidal thoughts during medical school. Medical students were also found to be 2-5 times more likely to have depression compared to general population. It is important to mention that this research done on a sample of 129,000 medical students in 47 countries, demonstrating the pervasiveness of the problem.

Unfortunately, only 16% of medical students who screened positive actually saw someone to discuss this problem.

This can be attributed to the fact that medical school training and studying is very stressful and competitive [1]. Students don't have time to take care of themselves or may fear that they are seen as less capable.

The Washington Post published an article entitled, "Medical school can be brutal, and it's making many of us suicidal" [2]. This report divulged the unexpected suicide of a well-preforming student and discussed reasons for the increased prevalence of suicide among medical students.

Academic competition is believed to be a main reason for the increased prevalence of suicide among medical students. In 2015, the average medical school accepted only 6.9% of applicants. Mayo Clinic had an even lower acceptance rate of 1.8%. This demonstrates the significant competition applicants go through to be accepted into medical school, and the sense of inadequacy applicants may feel if they do not get accepted or are not able to join the program of their choice.

Once in medical school, the stress continues. A medical student must study large quantities of material in very short periods of time, go through frequent exams, while competing with the best and smartest students. Failures and low scores are all reported in what is called the Dean's letter. The Dean's letter accompanies all applications the student submits for residency training. Having a bad Dean's letter can make it hard for the medical student to continue to pursue a career in medicine.

The medical student has to finish the United States Medical Licensing Exams (USMLE) or equivalent exams. There are 4 exams in total. Step 1 and step 2, each lasting 8 hours with about 50 questions per one-hour block. Then, step 2 clinical knowledge (CS), a simulation exam on patient actors, then step 3 which is a total of 16 hours—8 hours in 2 days. These exams are very difficult, stressful, and need considerable preparation and studying. So, in addition to the regular stressors of anxiety, lack of sleep, fatigue and worrying, these exams have the following problems:

1. If a student scores low in one exam, they cannot repeat the exam within seven years, so the student is stuck with this low score. Low scores sometimes will make it hard for the student to match for residency programs and can make it impossible to match for one of the top specialties. Therefore, one low exam score can crush the dream of being an orthopedic or a neurosurgeon.

2. Students have to follow two curricula: typical medical school courses and separate classes necessary for USMLE exams. Not only does this dissonance create distraction, but it also costs money

In addition to academic challenges, some students reported experiencing humiliation at the hands of senior clinicians during their first clinical rotations. Research demonstrates 80% of medical students have been mistreated by their supervisors. This can create a hostile learning environment.

I have seen students who on top of the stress of medical school also had social stressors. This can include issues with family or friends, or complications in their marriage. Maintaining relationships while in medical school can be complicated due to the competing demands for time. Stress at school and home can have negative effects and can worsen depression or suicidal thoughts.

Financial pressures can also increase stress. Every year, about 20,000 students will join medical school. On average, they will pay 50,000 USD per year or more. The average debt at graduation is 170,000 USD. Some publications showed that after calculating lost wages and accounting for tuition, it costs more than one million USD to graduate medical school. This high cost is calculated with the assumption a student will finish medical school on time with no obstacles or breaks during medical school, which is not always the case.

Is becoming a physician worth $2.6 million [3]?

Being under stress in medical school not only increases the risk of depression and suicide, but can also lead to sleep disorders, decreased concentration, increased incidence of errors, use of drugs and alcohol, and physical illnesses such as headache, heart diseases, and gastrointestinal diseases [4].

In addition to all that was discussed, the daily life of medical students can be very rough. For example, some universities will not have on-campus parking, often causing students to rely on public transportation to arrive promptly to their training location. This can be difficult if you need to arrive before public transportation starts running. It is not uncommon for medical students to arrive before 5am in order to prepare for the day.

With all what was mentioned, anyone can easily make the conclusion that being in medical school will also impact students' social life. I believe medical students have much less time to socialize compared to students of other schools.

Simply, admittance to medical school is competitive, stressful, requires very hard work, is expensive, impacts their social life, and predisposes them to an increased risk of depression and suicide. Throughout the rest of this book, I will continue to discuss the challenges encountered by aspiring physicians.

I received my medical school education in Egypt which follows the British system. We enter 7-8 years of an extended medical school right after finishing high school, followed by a mandatory internship. During our first year of medical school, only about 60 of the 300 students managed to pass all of their classes. Just as surprising, only 180 students in my class of 300 graduated on time I always maintained a high rank in medical school, but this required very long hours of study every single day. Looking back, I sacrificed my social life like many of my colleagues. Our time was almost entirely dedicated to study; we did not socialize or hang out with friends as much as colleagues in other careers did.

Medical school has its challenges all over the world. Articles illustrate the common trend is a need to study for long hours to remain competitive, and this comes at a price, particularly for people who desire to remain at the top of their class. Being at the top requires even more work, longer hours, and is very stressful to maintain the highest rank in order to enter the top specialties.

For students like me who graduated medical school in a foreign country, there are additional obstacles to practicing in the United States. First, foreign medical graduates are required to pass the USMLE exams. The challenge here is the style of the exams can be totally different than the style of exams in other countries. Learning the new style requires more training from the foreign medical graduate to be able to adapt to the new exam style. That will add more years after medical school studying for the USMLE exams, taking courses, and finally taking the exam.

Then, foreign medical graduates will apply for residency competing with American graduates and other graduates from all over the world. It is known that small percent of foreign medical graduates will be able to find a residency training program.

Once the graduate is accepted into a training program, there is the challenge of accommodating to the new culture of patient care and learning the logistics of a different health system.

I was lucky that my medical school was in English, but many other countries will have medical school taught in their own language. In this case, the language barrier can present a tremendous obstacle to taking the exams and interacting with patients.

It is also important to note that foreign medical graduates will finish their medical school and do all this study and exams while they are either at their residency training or working as physicians in the community with very limited time to do so. I was studying for my USMLE exams while working as a faculty member at the university and studying for my master's degree, which was a requirement for me to continue my work at the university. Looking back, I do not know how I did it.

While there are exams that can be taken over seas through accredited exam centers, there are two exams that require coming to the US. As expected, applying for a visa and travelling to the exam is extremely costly. I have several friends, who, after finishing the two exams in Egypt were denied visa entry to the US to take the other exams. This example is unique to foreign medical school students. I witnessed the dreams of friends who hoped to become physicians in the US crash after their visit to the embassy and the denial of their visa application. I have friends who scored highly, but without a visa, scores do not matter.

This is a brief summary of what a foreign medical graduate will face logistically to work in the US—just more work on top of the regular effort.

References

1. Rotenstein LS, Ramos MA, Torre M, Segal JB, Peluso MJ, Guille C, Sen S, Mata DA. Prevalence of Depression, Depressive Symptoms, and Suicidal Ideation Among Medical Students: A Systematic Review and Meta-Analysis. JAMA. 2016 Dec 6;316(21):2214-2236.

2. Medical school can be brutal, and it's making many of us suicidal. https://www.washingtonpost.com/national/health-science/medical-school-can-be-brutal-and-its-making-many-of-us-suicidal/2016/10/07/faa1a14e-8a4c-11e6-875e2c1bfe943b66_story.html?noredirect=on&utm_term=.9eb93ea4a667

3. "Is Becoming a Doctor Worth $2.6 Million?" http://thehealthcareblog.com/blog/2014/11/20/is-becoming-a-doctor-worth-2-6-million/

4. Khan, Rida; Lin, Jamie S.; Mata, Douglas A. ". Addressing Depression and Suicide Among Physician Trainees" JAMA Psychiatry. 2015 August, 72 (8): 848.

5. O'Rourke, M; Hammond, S. "The Medical Student Stress Profile: a tool for stress audit in medical training". Medical Education. 2010, 27 (44): 1027–1037.

RESIDENCY TRAINING

Following medical school, students apply for residency in their field of interest. Available fields include surgery, neurosurgery, anesthesiology, ophthalmology, and more. The residency training duration varies between different specialties.

Residency training, in my opinion, is probably the most stressful time of any physician's training phases. The trainee will be caring for very sick patients, working long hours, evaluated on a daily basis, while having to study, go through several very difficult exams, be sleep deprived in certain rotations, and stay overnight in the hospital at least few times a month, while being expected to not make any errors. Due to the busy time in residency, residents are at high risk of sleep deprivation which eposes residents to same risks as discussed with medical students including cardiovascular diseases, gastrointestinal disorders, breast cancer, miscarriage, preterm labor [1].

It is known that sleep deprivation in medical residents can lead to medical errors. In the past, residents routinely worked more than 24 hours during their night call shift, and sometimes more than 30 hours. This was the practice for decades until recent years when regulations limited the number of hours residents work to avoid the risks associated with lack of sleep.

One of the common rotations residents do is the night float rotation, where the resident will spend about a month working night shifts. This was found to impair the circadian rhythm of sleep and may have negative impact on their performance [2-5]. A study found that after 24 hours of sustained wakefulness, hand-eye coordination declines to a level equal to blood alcohol level of 0.1% [2].

Many studies reported issues with performance in medical residents due to sleep deprivation. One study evaluated the residents' ability to identify EKG arrhythmias and it was found that errors were higher in residents who were sleep deprived as compared to residents who were well rested.

Another study found that residents take more time and make more errors during laparoscopic surgery after being on call the night before [6-8].

It has been reported that empathy declines during the first year of residency while anger, depression and fatigue increase [9]. Stress during residency has been attributed to three main categories.

1. Work related stress such as long work hours, sleep deprivation and staff conflicts;

2. Stressor of personal life such as conflicts with peers, family members, spouse, financial struggles and moving to a new city (which is very common as residents apply for residency spots and they get the ones they match for which is not uncommonly to be in a new city whether by choice or due to the match obligations);

3. Professional stressors such as dealing with patients, studying, teaching and other academic and clinical responsibilities [10].

These stressors will be even magnified for the borderline resident who is unable to keep up efficiently with the competing demands during residency. I have heard of residents committing suicide due to the overwhelming stress during their residency training, in addition to personal stressors.

Other colleagues of mine have experienced drug addiction in an effort to lower their stress, jeopardizing their medical career all together. On the extreme end of the spectrum, some medical residents experiencing addiction may overdose, causing respiratory depression and eventually death.

I cannot tell you enough about the bad experience my colleagues and I had knowing that one of our own was found dead due to drug overdose. We will live with the guilt of wondering if we could have done anything to notice his addiction, and in turn, save his life.

Another important stressor during residency training is the financial burden. Graduating medical school can leave medical students with very high debt to pay as we discussed before. A resident salary is between 40 and 50K USD. While this is the salary for many other professions, medical students face the unique burden of having to pay off a large debt while using their remaining salary for typical living expenses.

The problem is magnified if the resident is married or has a family to support. Some residents will pick up shifts to make extra money (moonlighting). While the extra money is nice, it often means working weekends and late shifts, which increases work hours and time away from family.

I remember when I was a resident, making my way to the call room—a room with nothing but a small bed. Considering I probably hadn't slept for over 20 hours at this point, I was excited to rest. However, my sleep would be interrupted by my pager, typically only an hour into sleep, forcing me to return to work. Put simply, emergencies do not come at convenient times when physicians are fully rested and prepared for the day.

During residency training there are both early morning and after work lectures. It is common to see several residents sleeping in their chairs or trying to fight falling asleep. The key is, try your best and keep going.

While I enjoyed my residency training and was able to perform very well, I witnessed colleagues who could not finish their training due to health issues that made them unable to perform with a lack of sleep.

In addition to attending classes, taking exams, and working with patients, residents are expected to perform quality improvement projects, participate in teaching medical students, attend lectures, and prepare journal clubs and grand rounds on weekly bases.

After the end of residency, each resident will take the board exam of their specialty. The board exam is designed differently between different specialties; it can be made of one written exam, written and oral exams, written and oral and practical exams, or other forms.

The board exam typically requires long hours of studying, taking courses, and possibly travelling to the exam center. Most of this preparation phase will happen during the final year of training, as the board exam is typically taken shortly after the end of the residency training.

Residents typically finish their training by the end of June, and the board exam will be shortly after. It is important to note that most residents will start their fellowship training or a permanent job by July, which means they must do the final preparation for the exam and start a new job at the same time.

The demands of a new job can include moving to a new city, learning a new electronic medical record system, seeing patients for the first time independently, taking on more responsibilities, and meeting new colleagues.

I believe this in itself is a big burden, and the timing for the board exam is very bad, as this is a very busy time for a graduating resident. Just the timing can predispose people to fail, due to the many things going on simultaneously

During residency and through the medical career, any error will be investigated and presented in what we call the M & M (Mortality and Morbidity) meeting where a faculty will present all the mistakes and errors that happened during the month. Sometimes the resident who made the error will be asked to present their own error.

While the goal of this meeting is educational, and the information should be used for quality improvement, in some institutes it becomes a humiliating event. The person involved may feel criticized and people may gossip about the resident who made the error.

It is not uncommon that a resident will quit residency due to a myriad of factors. Reasons for leaving residency may include bullying, burnout, anxiety, disenchantment, concerns about the future of medicine, and more.

While quitting can be the right decision, residents who quit will have now all the medical school and undergraduate education loans to pay off. However, it is still better to quit at this point before it is too late.

References

1. See Biological Rhythms: Implications for the Worker, publication OTA-BA-463 (U.S. Congress, Office of Technology Assessment, 1991); Bøggild Henrik, Knutsson Anders (1999). "Shift Work, Risk Factors, and Cardiovascular Disease". Scandinavian Journal of Work and Environmental Health. 25 (2): 85–99.

2. Dawson, Drew; Reid, Kathryn. Fatigue, alcohol and performance impairment. Nature. 1997 July, 388 (6639): 235–235. (https://www.nature.com/articles/40775).

3. Bolster, Lauren; Rourke, Liam. "The Effect of Restricting Residents' Duty Hours on Patient Safety, Resident Well-Being, and Resident Education: An Updated Systematic Review". Journal of Graduate Medical Education. 2015, 7 (3): 349–363.

4. Cavallo, Anita; Ris, M. Douglas; Succop, Paul. "The night float paradigm to decrease sleep deprivation: good solution or a new problem? Ergonomics. 2003, 46(7): 653–663.

5. Landrigan, Christopher P.; Rothschild, Jeffrey M.; Cronin, John W.; Kaushal, Rainu; Burdick, Elisabeth; Katz, Joel T.; Lilly, Craig M.; Stone, Peter H.; Lockley, Steven W.; Bates, David W.; Czeisler, Charles A. "Effect of Reducing Interns' Work Hours on Serious Medical Errors in Intensive Care Units". New England Journal of Medicine. 2004, 351 (18): 1838–1848.

6. Smith-Coggins R, Rosekind MR, Buccino KR. Relationship of day versus night sleep to physician performance and mood. Ann Emerg Med 1994; 24:928-934.

7. Friedman RC, Bigger JT, Kornfeld DS. The intern and sleep loss. N Eng J Med 1971; 285:201-203.

8. Taffinder NJ, McManus IC, Gul Y, et al. Effect of sleep deprivation on surgeons' dexterity on laparoscopy simulator Lancet 1998; 352:1191.

9. Bellini LM, Baime M, Shea JA. Variation of mood and empathy during internship. JAMA. 2002; 287:3143–3146

10. Levey RE. Sources of stress for residents and recommendations for programs to assist them. Acad Med. 2001; 76:142–150.

FELLOWSHIP TRAINING

After the end of residency, a resident can choose to start working in their chosen field or go on to further training for sub specialization. For example, graduating from Anesthesiology training, a resident can choose to practice as a general anesthesiologist or continue onto a fellowship in several subspecialties such as Pain Medicine (which I did), cardiac anesthesiology (to become an expert in providing Anesthesia during heart surgeries), Pediatric Anesthesiology (to be able to provide Anesthesia for children) and more.

Some subspecialties require 2 fellowships, for example pediatric cardiac anesthesiology will require extra training focused on providing anesthesia for open heart surgery for children. So, the resident will perform a pediatric anesthesia fellowship followed by a pediatric cardiac anesthesia fellowship. In some subspecialties, the training can be even more extensive.

The length of fellowship training varies between different subspecialties. Most fellowships range between 1 and 3 years in length. Depending on the subspecialties chosen, this means to complete medical school residency, and fellowship training can amount to 11 years or more.

The stressors of residency are similar to the challenges faced in fellowship. However, in my opinion, fellowship is less stressful if you had good clinical experiences in residency because of the increase in competence and knowledge.

A benefit is that if a fellow decides to leave the fellowship, they are still able to practice the main specialty they trained on during residency. In addition, they can still obtain board certification for their primary residency. Residents on the other hand, if terminated from residency, will most likely not be able to practice medicine again. In addition, there is a slight increase in salary and in some instances (not always), better work hours.

Each fellowship typically will require the fellow to take a board exam specific for each subspecialty. For those with multiple subspecialties, this may mean more than 1 board exam.

When I was making the decision about completing a fellowship, one of my colleagues who did not do a fellowship told me: doing a fellowship is like watching your favorite car leaving your drive way. My colleague was referring to the fact that you lose the salary of a physician for one or more years during the fellowship, which could buy a luxurious car had it not been pursued.

While it would be assumed that fellowship trained physicians would make more money, this is actually not always the case. In many instances, fellowship trained physicians can make similar salaries as those who did not pursue a fellowship. On the other hand, fellowship training can improve job market and opportunities, yet again this is not guaranteed.

To reiterate, for many physicians, a fellowship is not about the money or status, rather it is out of genuine interest. If the candidate is interested in a subspecialty, then a fellowship is required and should be pursued.

DO PHYSICIANS MAKE
ENOUGH MONEY?

While many people believe all physicians have high salaries, this is not true.

Let us first make a calculation. It takes a minimum of 11-14 years in higher education to become a physician. If you choose to complete a PhD, MPH, and/or MBA, training will be even longer. During those years, the aspiring physician will be accumulating loans for undergraduate and medical school (and more for MPH, Masters or other extra studies), while not producing any income. Students who go to medical school are high achievers but let's assume a hypothetical student would decide not to pursue medical school. They would receive an average job with an income of 50,000 USD per year. This equates to the student losing the opportunity to make a minimum of 500,000 USD per year by not working during the time they'd spend becoming a physician.

The average loan for a medical student is 166,750 USD, and if paid at 7.5 % rate over 30 years, the total debt will be 419,738 USD. These numbers are very conservative. Some undergraduate and medical schools, especially out of state or private colleges will be much more expensive, which can double or triple the amount of debt.

Therefore, going to medical school to become a physician is called by some the one-million-dollar mistake (it can be the 2 or 3 million mistake for others!).

During residency and fellowship training salaries are a 40,000-70,000 USD per year. During this time interest on student loans continues to accrue. Fellowship, with this low salary, can continue for more than 10 years while training is completed.

Once you complete residency and fellowship there is a lot of variation among salaries of practicing physician. Depending on the location and institution, an average salary is around 100,000 USD. Currently Family Medicine and Internal Medicine are among the lowest paid specialties, despite their very important role in caring for the health of the population. Therefore, although people may believe that physicians make exorbitant amounts of money, it is not the case for many physicians. One day, I looked up the list of the richest people in the world, and believe me, none of them is a physician.

It is also important to note that the average physician income has been declining over the years and continues to decline. Some reports showed that the average physician's take home pay is less than 28 USD per day in some cases.

While many people are under the impression that physicians' salaries are the main cause of our high health spending in the United States, this is a total misconception. Physician salaries represent 20% of national health care spending, and about 10% of this amount goes into physician practice expenses, as malpractice insurance and other similar expenses. The reality is physicians' salaries make up 10% of total national health care spending.

There have been proposals to decrease physician's salaries by 20%, to aid high healthcare costs. I feel this would be a poor choice. Physicians have sacrificed their 20's and 30's to become providers of healthcare, while accruing significant amounts of debt. Cutting physician salaries by 20% would only reduce the total national health spending by only 2% [1] and would likely discourage many potential candidates from even entering the profession. Would this really be worth the risk of losing high quality candidates?

Another interesting report looked at the cost of study, time spent not working, and average salaries for different physician specialties and developed a formula to calculate the return investment of being in different specialties. They discovered that primary care providers and pediatricians have a negative net return value, meaning they are a poor return on investment, yet these are some of the most important specialties. Primary care providers and pediatricians represent a main corner stone in our health care system as they are the go-to providers for many health issues. They provide thorough evaluations, guide patients to appropriate treatments, and work to improve the health of the population. Primary care providers are also the ones who determine whether a referral to a subspecialty is needed, can diagnose serious diseases early on, and are the gate to our health care system [2].

There was another interesting report that compared how much physicians make during their career versus teachers. The authors looked at average

26

years of study, lost wages, and final salary (based on the assumption the student will not have any issues during their career course), and the results were shocking. The authors concluded that physicians make 3 cents less per hour than high school teachers over the course of their career.

Again, this gap could be much larger if the student studies for more years, completes longer training for sub specialization, repeats a semester, or takes any breaks [4].

Therefore, when you think about becoming a physician, you may see the years of hard study and believe it pays well at the end, but in many instances, that is not the case.

There are many other career opportunities that allow people to make significantly more money than physicians, and to have a nicer lifestyle with substantially less stress. Therefore, money should never be the motivation for anyone to go to medical school.

Reimbursement for health services is declining every year, which in turn will also likely impact a physician's future salary. If insurance companies are paying less, then salaries will be less. With recent reforms in health care, more patients are covered by government healthcare program which typically provide lower reimbursement to health systems, and therefore to physicians.

This is a major worry. If reimbursements keep declining, and in turn physicians' salaries become lower, this will create more financial stress on physicians. Education costs historically have been increasing significantly and with low salaries it will be difficult to keep up with paying education loans.

This will also make medicine a less attractive career, just based on the financial stress alone. Let us think of the worst scenario here. A student will go out of state for undergraduate, attend a prestigious and expensive medical school, and then become a physician in one of the many low paying specialties. This will be a huge problem as it will be extremely hard to pay off massive student loans with a low salary.

I am referring to our nation's current situation, but current trends predict that education will become more expensive, and salaries will continue to decline. Therefore, the current financial stressors are expected to only get worse.

I would like to also bring to the reader's attention that we talked in depth about loans and salaries. However, there are other financial stressors that a physician can encounter, including and not limited to, the money a physician may have to spend if sued by a patient. Some cases settle for a quarter of a million dollars or more, even if the physician was not found guilty. That is why physicians pay liability insurance, even though it can be very expensive for some specialties like obstetrics and gynecology.

Obstetricians (physicians whom specialize in childbirth) will typically pay for malpractice insurance for several years after retirement as each child they deliver has the ability to sue them for a certain number of years after delivery, typically around 18 years of age.

We as a nation should be weary of declining physician salaries and increasing health care and education costs. It has been estimated that we will be short 20,000 primary care providers by 2020 [3].

References

1. Doctors make far less money than most people think. https://www.kevinmd.com/blog/2010/06/doctors-money-people.html

2. How does your salary stack up against various medical specialties? https://www.statnews.com/2017/07/18/doctors-salary-specialties/

3. https://bhw.hrsa.gov/health-workforce-analysis/primary-care-2020

4. The Deceptive Salary of Doctors – BestMedicalDegrees.com https://www.bestmedicaldegrees.com/salary-of-doctors/

PHYSICIANS' SOCIAL LIFE

After many years of training, and officially becoming a physician, many believe this is when life finally begins. But soon after starting the job, the new physician will discover that this is not as they thought. Physicians encounter many problems in their career that can significantly impact their life outside of the job.

The first issue I will discuss is the impact of being a physician on our social life. The medical profession will require a physician spend long hours at work (the amount varies between different specialties) that may consume all the physician's energy. Part of this is that physicians cannot say no to any patient, as doing so is ethically wrong. So as long as there are patients, there is more work to be done.

Seeing a plethora of patients for widespread reasons leaves a physician drained at the end of the workday, as you are required to put forth your best effort forth for every patient. After, when you go home, you're expected to be involved with one's family and kids (if you have decided to start one) and be able to socialize with friends. The demands of a medical career leave a physician's social life difficult to keep up with.

It is important to note that even after going home, the work day is not over. Many times, the physician sees so many patients during the day, they spend their evenings typing up their notes. In addition, many physicians are also responsible for responding to calls they get from patients after hours, depending on the specialty or work location. Calls can happen at any time, even in the middle of the night during much needed rest.

There are some things a physician can do to balance time in order to socialize and have a somewhat normal family life. One thing that many physicians do is to function as a part of a team, so one team member is on call every week. This may not be an option for solo practitioners, or those who own their practice and have no partners. It is important not to try to be a superhero and do too much but rather, a physician needs to take breaks and pace themselves. Physicians should have hobbies they enjoy and try to find a dedicated time to practice these hobbies. They need to be in touch with family and friends as much as they can and be involved in social events. A physician should ask for help at work if the situation is beyond his/her clinical skills, and socially by seeing a counselor to improve coping skills which can help them balance work, family, and social life.

I would like to share with you a personal story to show you how much we miss out on in our social lives. I have a friend who one day went home, and his little daughter said "daddy" to him. My friend was ecstatic and immediately called his wife over and told her that their daughter had finally started talking. The wife looked at him and told him, "honey she has been talking for three weeks now."

My friend was extremely disappointed, and he immediately recognized it was time for a change. He reduced his work hours so he could go home earlier and spend more time with his family. This decision impacted him financially, but he felt it was important to prioritize family over money, as moments like this in our lives are priceless. On the other hand, this was not beneficial for his patients as they now have to wait longer to receive his care, a problem that will be discussed later in this book.

Another friend of mine who specialized in neurosurgery worked extensive hours during his training. He told me that his oldest daughter treated him as a stranger for the first 2 years of her life. She treated him like someone she would briefly see in and out of her home, not recognizing that this was her father.

I know of a couple where both the husband and wife are physicians and were in training together. They worked long hours, so they relied on a nanny to help them raise their child. My friends told me that after a while, the daughter thought the nanny was her mother and she was more attached to her than her own parents. This was an absolute awful feeling as described by my friends.

Research shows it is harder on the child when both parents are away. I also worry about the lack of normal support a child requires from at least one consistent parent in their life. This can greatly impact the future relationship between the parents and their children. The reason I am proposing this hypothesis is I have seen kids who have lost attachment to their physician parent as they were always away, and as a result healthy relationship was not cultivated.

Another common issue that physicians encounter is getting paged while on call and having to go to the hospital immediately. It is common that we get paged when we are spending time with family, attending social events, or even our kids' activities and parties. Given physicians will have many days and night of call over the years, it is likely that all physicians will experience this in their career.

I had my daughter when I was still in my residency training when I was busy with work, studying, and taking my board exams. I finished my training when she was 2 years old, and I did my best during that time to spend as much time with her as I could, as time for me was so limited. I had my son when I was a faculty member, so I definitely had more time to be a part of raising him, as compared to when I was a resident. Seeing my son grow in his first 2 years showed me how much I missed with my daughter, and just how many milestones I missed with her because I was not around as much.

I became very aware that I needed to spend and dedicate more time with my kids and try not to miss their important events, when possible. While I try hard, I still miss out on things due to the lack of flexibility in my schedule. When I am with my children, I try to be present in the moment to the best extent I can, as I know they will leave home one day. My greatest hope is not to have any regrets about the time I didn't spend with them, by making the moments I can count.

It is very important for physicians to be aware of their work-life balance. In some specialties, physicians will routinely leave the hospital at 8 pm, usually arriving home when their kids are in bed. It is not uncommon that I hear from colleagues that days will go by without seeing their kids due to the early morning start and late-night end of the work day.

During residency training and afterwards, some physicians will be required to work in the hospital on holidays and weekends. Therefore, it is common for the physician to miss important holidays, family gatherings, and kids' events. Regardless, someone must be in the hospital at all times to care for the patients.

It is important to realize that hospitals cannot close. If I wake up one day and there is a severe snow storm, schools will close, companies will close, but hospitals must stay open which means physicians must make their way to the hospital somehow. I do not believe that there is a solution to this, as it is the nature of the job, and extreme weather is even more reason for hospitals and physicians to be available.

In certain specialties, physicians spend many nights in the hospital, going home the following morning, usually sleeping all day and then going back to work at night. This is very typical for emergency department physicians. When working the night shift, it is challenging to participate in any family activities due to the nature of the hours and the sleep disturbances that will typically occur.

PHYSICIANS AND RELATIONSHIPS

Some spouses and children of physicians have the ability to live a high-status lifestyle, especially if the physician is in a high salary specialty. While many believe that the family life of a physician is ideal, investigators found that the stress in the physician's life can be damaging to family life, their children, and marital partners, regardless of their pay.

Another study assessing physicians' stress indicated that marriage and sexual relationships for physicians are often unsatisfactory. Physicians are at risk for developing emotional separation from family, especially in the early years of their career which then becomes an important factor leading to divorce [1].

While there are several stressors that impact physicians, a majority stems from emotional stress. Physicians constantly deal with sick patients, make decisions related to life and death, have high expectations from patients and their families, while trying to work within organizational and insurance constraints. In the midst of all these responsibilities, the physician's family may be ignored, which can lead to family issues.

A physician's job requires accuracy and precision, and this may reflect on their expectations for their family members. Expecting perfection at home can create a gap between the physician and their spouse and children.

Physicians also tend to deny they are affected by emotional and social stressors and are less likely to ask for help, which in turn can worsen their emotional and social problems. This further creates more problems in their relationships.

It has been reported that for female physicians, the pressure is even greater. Female physicians are typically high achievers and set very high expectations for themselves. With such success, any inability to perform any tasks, such as child care, can be considered by them a failure.

Equity in the medical filed is very important. A study performed on 85 women physicians found that one third of them had no domestic help; 75 % of them did their own cooking, shopping, financial management and child care. It has been reported that some female physicians marry other physicians who understand the nature and the demand of the career.

Seemingly, it was found that they tend to help less with daily activities. These factors create even more pressure and stress on women physicians due to the many competing demands both in the work place and at home.

Patients may feel abandoned when their physician becomes pregnant or turn to a part time schedule. Unfortunately, this situation can also be perceived poorly by colleagues and partners who should be more understanding.

It is a shame that medical schools do not teach students about their self-care and the importance of keeping a work life balance. Physicians are devoted to their patients and their career, but they need to be reminded that they are human too.

The problem starts in medical school. Most medical students are academically focused, competitive, and hardworking, understanding there is no room for error [1].

When you think about who the common role models for medical students are, you will recognize that they are often physicians with impressive research achievements, internationally known physicians, and clinicians who spend long hours caring for patients. Many of those role models live a life extremely out of balance. This may lead medical students believe this is what is needed to succeed.

The "ideal" characteristic for a physician include self-control, hard long hours of work, dedication, and perfectionism, which are all traits that are counterintuitive to creating healthy relationships and marriages [2].

There are other factors that can make physicians' relationships very challenging. Those factors include working in rural areas where a lack of physicians may mean longer work hours and require being on call more frequently. This is not only hard on the physician but can be very demanding on their relationships with their spouses and children. Physicians who perform locums (per diem jobs) may have to travel a majority of the time, leaving their family to travel for the job assignment location which can be several hours away from home.

In especially challenging specialties like obstetrics and neurosurgery, physicians have very little control over their time, often working long hours and can be called at any time of the day and night.

Due to the massive debt physicians acquire while in school, many pick up more calls and shifts to be able to pay these debts. This leads to even more hours of work which is often over night or on weekends which. This increase in work hours reduces the time they spend with their family members.

On the other hand, physicians who are able to maintain good work-life balance are happier. Unfortunately, in order to achieve this, they may have to work less, which can impact their income and may create stress of another nature.

Research indicates it is not uncommon for physicians to come from difficult childhoods, which for many can be a strong motivator to pursue a career as a physician. Many experienced very difficult life situations such as poverty, hunger, or forced migration. Other have experienced discrimination, abuse, or disease. These experiences may create resilience and strength but come with their emotional and physical challenges [3].

Physicians who come from families that suffered divorce may have a fear of marriage and relationships, which increases their risk of family discord [4].

Some training programs are very toxic which can make the trainee unable to create and maintain a normal relationship with others.

We have not talked about other family relations, such as relationships with parents, siblings, and friends. In my opinion, during the residency training, those relationships will significantly decline due to the many competing demands, particularly if the family and friends live in a different state.

In my case, my family lives overseas and I could not travel at all during my residency training. When my parents, God bless their heart, came to visit me, I was only able to take one week off to spend time with them. I then had to be back to work for the rest of their stay. When I was back working, they would see me for about only 4 hours at night. During those 4 hours, I was extremely exhausted and may have been studying as well. It is a difficult feeling when you have your loved ones whom you have not seen

38

for several years living in your home, yet you still cannot spend much time with them.

My parents' visits during my residency training showed me the incredible love parents have for their kids. Staying in my small apartment, trying to have dinner prepared by the time I am home, and spending only brief time with me each day. For them, the visit must have been quite boring, as they were stuck inside the apartment because they were dependent on me to take them out, which happened infrequently because I was busy working.

References

1. Dickstein LJ. Medical students and residents: issues and needs. In: Goldman LS, Myers M, Dickstein LJ, eds. *The Handbook of Physician Health.* Chicago: American Medical Association; 2000:161-179.

2. Ellis JJ, Inbody DR. Psychotherapy with physicians' families: when attributes in medical practice become liabilities in family life. *Am J Psychother* 1988; 42:380-388.

3. Myers MF. Physicians and intimate relationships. In: Goldman LS, Myers M, Dickstein LJ, eds. *The Handbook of Physician Health.* Chicago: American Medical Association; 2000: 52-79.

4. Myers MF. *Intimate Relationships in Medical School: How to Make Them Work.* Thousand Oaks, CA: Sage Publications; 2000.

PHYSICIANS AND DIVORCE

Physicians work long hours and are under constant stress. Previous research suggests physicians have a higher divorce rate compared to non-physicians [1-3], however a recent review of the literature shows mixed results on this topic.

A study done on this issue 40 years ago showed that physicians have a markedly higher divorce rate compared to non-physician. The study also related poor self-rated marriages. However, this study was limited due to small sample size [4].

There was another interesting study performed on 1118 medical graduates from Johns Hopkins University in 1997. The results of this study indicated that the divorce rate among medical graduates was 29 %. Psychiatrists and surgeons had the highest divorce rates (50% and 33% respectively) [5].

While those 2 studies provide evidence that divorce among physicians was higher than other professions, they had several limitations and their results are hard to generalize.

A national survey conducted that used data between 1970 and 1980 found different results. The Survey indicated that physicians have a similar divorce rate to other professionals [6]. Based on this data, it is difficult to make a conclusion, but it is evident that physicians will have more family problems than others even if it does not reach the point of divorce.

It is also important that most of those studies were performed decades ago. The rate of divorce in the United States has also decreased overall.

While the results are conflicting, literature proposed that female physicians and females working in healthcare are more likely to go through divorce as compared to women in other professions. Reasons for this are that female physicians often carry a larger burden, as they provide more care for their family and children which creates more stress in addition to their long days at work.

Some surveys also proposed that physicians typically marry at a later age, so they have fewer years of marriage and that is why their divorce rate might seem similar to non-physicians.

In my opinion, the physician has to take careful consideration with their life partner. It is important to choose a partner who will understand their career challenges, stresses and time demand, and be willing to support their physician partner. I read online that the main reason why physicians divorced was because their spouses did not recognize the career demand and the long hours, they work which created family stress and led to the end of the marriage.

Some people marry a physician thinking they will have an easy life, good income, and enjoyable lifestyle. As I have shown, this is not typically the case.

I have also read about extreme cases that did not end in divorce, but rather with suicide or even homicide. In some instances, one spouse kills the other and then commits suicide. There are many devastating stories in the news throughout the years that show how important it is to choose the right person when you have a demanding career.

References

1. Myers MF. The well-being of physician relationships. West J Med 2001; 174:30–3.

2. Derdeyn AP. The physician's work and marriage. Int J Psychiatry Med 1978; 9:297–306.

3. Rose KD, Rosow I. Marital stability among physicians. Calif Med 1972; 116:95–9.

4. Vaillant GE, Sobowale NC, McArthur C. Some psychologic vulnerabilities of physicians. N Engl J Med 1972; 287:372–5.

5. Rollman BL, Mead LA, Wang NY, Klag MJ. Medical specialty and the incidence of divorce. N Engl J Med 1997; 336:800–3.

6. Doherty WJ, Burge SK. Divorce among physicians. Comparisons with other occupational groups. JAMA 1989; 261:2374–7.

PATIENTS' COMPLAINTS

Patients may become dissatisfied with their physician for many reasons, both logical and illogical. Therefore, it is important that patients provide feedback if they feel the physician is not performing up to their standards, is mistreating them, or for any other serious concerns. Unfortunately, sometimes patients complain because the physician did not agree with them or provided medical advice that the patient did not like.

When unhappy patients may react differently. Some will not discuss it, some will request another provider, and some will take action of varying degrees [1-3].

Actions a patient may take include reporting the physician to the hospital or medical group, complaining to the state medical board, filing a claim and taking the case to court, or even submitting a grievance to the state medical society. In addition, some patients will take more than one action against a physician.

Outside of the medical field, people can always complain to a manager, or call customer service to file a complaint. Many people believe the adage "the customer is always right" and take full advantage of their right to complain.

An interesting study indicated that the majority of grievances are filed by younger women against newly encountered physicians. The main reason found for the complaints was a lack of communication [4].

Another study indicated that the most common reasons for disagreement between a patient and their physician is failure to make a diagnosis, disagreement about a prescription, concern over the interaction, and alleged over or under treatment [5].

In my opinion, patients' complaints mainly stem from the failure of the physician and the health system to meet their expectations. Physicians are limited by many external forces; they have to follow national, state, societal, and hospital guidelines while ensuring they follow personal and ethical standards. The work demands paperwork, documentation, and the need to see too many patients in a limited amount of time. Many physicians are pressured to reduce wait times so patients can be seen in a timely manner, which means less time with each patient. Imagine seeing a new patient who comes to you with multiple concerns, and you are given 20 minutes to take their history, perform an evaluation and come up with a thorough diagnosis and treatment plan.

Some examples from my experience: a patient with a 10:30 am appointment shows up at 10:45 am, and by the time the patient is checked in and vital signs are taken, it is 10:55 am. The physician has another patient scheduled at 11 am. The physician cannot ethically deny seeing the first patient (physicians typically cannot say NO) so they will have to rush this visit, to be able to see the next patient who hopefully showed up on time. It is not uncommon that the patient that showed up late will complain that his/her visit was rushed, and the physician was not thorough in his/her exam.

Some patients will not show up for their visits time after time. After many no shows the provider may choose to no longer see them, and then the patient can file a complaint and the provider may have to accept them back as a patient again. The problem with no shows is that it reduces access to everyone. The spot that was not utilized by the patient who did not show up could been filled by another patient who instead might have to wait a few months to be seen. This is not cost effective for the health system since there are several logistical and cost considerations around each appointment.

I am not trying to undermine patients' experiences, as understanding the patient view point is extremely important and most definitely encouraged. Reporting concerns is needed to improve the medical field.

If the complaint took a legal route and was filed with the state medical board or in the court system, it may lead to countless hours of additional work from the physician to respond, and extreme stress and anxiety. This will not only impact the physician but may also affect their ability to provide excellent patient care to their other patients. It may even cause the physician to leave the profession entirely.

Again, patients' complaints and feedback are highly necessary to enhance clinical practice and improve the performance of physicians, however complaints should be valid and honest, if they are going to be beneficial in improving care.

47

In some cases, the complainant is not the patient, rather a significant other or family member. The physician needs to be aware family dynamics and include the family in discussions and decision making as appropriate. This is good practice and, in most cases, will keep the family happy, but for some challenging patients or family members it can be an impossible demand.

On television I see advertisements from law firms asking patients to call them if they had a bad outcome from a healthcare experience. If the patient calls, they may be encouraged to file a law suit against their physicians or possibly even the entire health system that treated them. We see this on TV, and displayed on big billboards on the highway, and we think it is a good thing. Unfortunately, this culture of litigation increases medical costs and has not been shown to improve quality of care. This practice of mass advertising to find people to file medical lawsuits is illegal in other countries, where lawyers are not able to make these kinds of advertisements. Again, if the concern is valid and serious, taking it to court might be the appropriate action.

I have a friend, who heard a patient talking to her boyfriend on the phone saying "...honey, these guys know what they are doing, we will not be able to sue them." It became apparent the patient was in the hospital that day to find a way to sue her physician to make money.

Again, I am not saying the majority of patients are doing this, actually this is done by fewer patients. Patients have the right and need to complain if they have a legitimate reason. Concerns such as malpractice and abuse have to be taken very seriously, as this is a breach of the Hippocratic Oath. Complaints have led to discovery of poor behaviors by some physicians which led to correction and reprimand. However, a minority of patients will abuse this and see it as a potential source of income, which is inappropriate.

I have known colleagues who ended up leaving the USA to practice in other countries due to the many complaints they had, and the settlements they had to pay (in millions sometimes) due to errors that can be attributed to system errors rather than personal errors.

References

1. Annandale E, Hunt K. Accounts of disagreements with doctors. Soc Sci Med 1998; 46:119-129.

2. Kravitz RL, Callahan EJ, Paterniti D, Antonius D, Dunham M, Lewis CE. Prevalence and sources of patients' unmet expectations for care. Ann Intern Med 1996; 125:730-737.

3. Klein R. Complaints Against Doctors. London: Charles Knight; 1973.

4. Halperin EC. Grievances against physicians: 11 years' experience of a medical society grievance committee. West J Med. 2000 Oct;173(4):235-8.

5. Annandale E, Hunt K. Accounts of disagreements with doctors. Soc Sci Med 1998; 46:119-129.

BEING UNDER INVESTIGATION

Physicians are frequently investigated, leading to it becoming a routine process in the medical field. An investigation can be initiated by anyone: patient, nurse, colleague. Literally anyone can complain for any reason and the physician will be placed under investigation. The seriousness of the investigation varies from something as simple as a need for quality improvement, to something more serious such as an error that led to a patient death. No matter the reason, the process is usually long, time consuming, and very stressful.

Investigations can run at the institutional, state and/or federal level. Even if the physician and complainant decide to settle the case, it will be still reported in national databases and may impact the physician when they apply for jobs or another state license in the future.

In the UK in 2014, there were 2750 General Medical Counsel (GMC) investigations launched. Several of those physicians under investigation complained about the stress this process causes and the feeling of being guilty until proven otherwise. Between 2005 and 2013, 28 physicians with open GMC investigations committed suicide [1].

It has also been noted in the UK that the number of patient complaints against physicians is increasing, doubling from 2007 to 2012. A large reason for this increase was due to the media [2-4].

In a large survey in the UK, investigators sent a survey to 95,636 physicians with a 11.4 % response rate. Of these, 6,146 had a previous or current complaint. Investigators analyzed the physicians' answers about the impact of the complaint and being under investigation.

Physicians reported feeling powerless, distressed, and described other negative feelings. Physicians were stressed because of the length of the process, the unpredictability of the outcomes and the worries about bias towards the patient. Some physicians reported finding a different career [5].

Even if the physician is innocent, it is very stressful, costs a lot of time and money, and the media may make a "good" story out of it. This will destroy the physician's reputation, family and social life, and may impact their future practice. Even their children may be impacted, by being the son or the daughter of a physician who was on the news.

Stories covered by media remain online, and even if the physician is proven to be innocent in the end, the damage has been done and is hard to reverse.

While there are several published articles on the stress physicians go through while under investigation in the UK and other counties, there is very little published in the US.

Investigations represent another stressor that physicians have to deal with. The problem is that investigations are becoming more common and are often based on a difference of opinion rather than true malpractice.

Best-case scenario, the physician is cleared or the case is closed due to a lack of evidence. Regardless of the outcome, if a physician undergoes more than one investigation in their career, it translates to few years of stress and can be for unfounded reasons.

If the investigation takes years, or leads to federal reporting, it may cause more stress for a longer duration regardless of the outcome. If the physician is guilty, then a penalty is appropriate.

I know physicians who left their job due to bad administration that did not protect their physicians from unfounded accusations. Some physicians consider leaving medicine, and some even commit suicide.

Even if the physician is found innocent, I believe it will still leave a scar and the physician may become overly cautious to avoid this experience again in the future. This may lead to changes in how they practice and interact with patients, staff, or colleagues.

References

1. Reducing stress for doctors undergoing an investigation – Medical professionalism and regulation in the UK https://gmcuk.wordpress.com/2016/01/13/reducing-stress-for-doctors-undergoing-an-investigation/

2. General Medical Council. The state of medical education and practice in the UK report: 2013. http://www.gmc-uk.org/publications/23435.asp.

3. General Medical Council. The state of medical education and practice in the UK report: 2014. 2014. http://www.gmc-uk.org/ publications/25452.asp.

4. General Medical Council. The state of medical education and practice in the UK report: 2015. 2015. http://www.gmc-uk.org/ publications/somep2015.asp

5. ourne T, Vanderhaegen J, Vranken R, Wynants L, De Cock B, Peters M, Timmerman D, Van Calster B, Jalmbrant M, Van Audenhove C. Doctors' experiences and their perception of the most stressful aspects of complaints processes in the UK: an analysis of qualitative survey data. BMJ Open. 2016 Jul 4;6(7): e011711.

DEALING WITH POLICIES
AND BUREAUCRACY

Healthcare is inundated with policies, guidelines and best practice recommendations, which all impact physician practice.

One study indicated that physicians spend at least 3 hours for documenting the quality of their care every week [1].

Studies demonstrate that access to physician appointments are a struggle all over the country. Part of the problem is that in the US a physician spends more than 22 % of their time on non-clinical paper work. This would be like removing 165,000 physicians from the workforce and having them only perform administrative work rather than seeing patients. And unfortunately, the situation is worsening, not improving [2].

Physicians in private practice have been expressing concern about several regulations that made their practices "die" over time. Recent regulations increased the costs associated with private practice, leading to many physicians closing or selling their practices. In 2005, two-thirds of the medical practices in the US were physician owned. Within 10 years, this number decreased to 50% [3].

Many regulations have been implemented in an effort to improve quality of care. Unfortunately, a significant number of these measures require countless hours of documentation by physicians, medical staff and administrators. While is it important to have quality metrics to ensure good care, these measures can be overly extensive, overwhelming, and may be not be helpful at improving outcomes. Many of these measures are also very subjective, making it difficult to assess the validity of the results.

Measures should be objective and reasonable to allow for actual improvement. Some payors such as the Centers for Medicaid and Medicare Services link payment incentives to the results of patient surveys and quality metrics. Hospitals are also moving toward taking these metrics into account when reimbursing their physicians.

While the idea is great in theory, the nature of the measures and implementation process is challenging.

Over the years, the amount of governance and oversight of every aspect of health care has increased. This requires physicians and health care systems to divert their time from patient care to paperwork. If the care is not appropriately documented, regardless of the quality of care provided, there are consequences.

A contributing factor for these problems is the dual governance over the health system by both state and federal organizations. This can lead to tension, especially when the standards are different, and cause further confusion for physicians and health systems.

I read an example that shows the different entities involved in the health care system. To practice medicine, a potential physician will attend medical school which is accredited by a private entity, take a national examination administered by a non-government entity, obtain a license to practice from the state medical board which is a government body, complete residency training which is funded by the government, obtain certification from a private organization, and then obtain privileges from a hospital which could be a private or public entity.

After achieving all of this, the physician legally is under the authority of the hospital they work for, which can be private or public, and also under the supervision of the state medical board, which belongs to the government [4].

Regulations not only impact the health system and physicians, but indirectly impact the patient. The large amount time spent documenting compliance with policies and regulations reduces the time for patient care. I am not proposing that we remove regulations, as they are essential for ensuring quality care, but the amount of documentation required to "prove" compliance and the measures themselves need to be streamlined to decrease the amount of paperwork.

In addition, the current regulations for approving medications requires pharmaceutical companies to perform extensive measures and clinical trials in order to have a new drug or device approved. Companies will encounter high costs during their work on this process and the end outcome is an expensive drug that patients cannot afford, and insurance companies will be reluctant to cover.

While this is a tough situation, on one side we want to make sure the drugs are well tested but on the other side, they need to be affordable. I do not have an answer for this one other than keeping a good balance. In other countries including Europe, the approval process is less tedious and less costly; it might be time to adopt new approaches.

Also, when it comes to insurance, there are the Governmental insurance (Medicare and Medicaid) and private insurance companies. Both entities follow different rules, have different reimbursement plans and values. They do not approve procedures or medications to the same degree. It is very common that an interventional procedure will be approved by one insurance entity and not by the others. There are also differences between the Governmental entities among each other and the same goes for private insurance companies among each other. Simply put, there is no common standard, and physicians and health care providers have to be aware of the differences between all payors.

Donald Berwick, former director of the Centers for Medicare and Medicaid Services, indicated that the needless administrative complexity led to about 107-389 billion dollars of waste in 2011. This waste resulted from lack of standard processes as standard form and similar.

The same insurance company will negotiate rates and coverage with a health system annually which makes the situation very complex as one system may deal with hundreds of payors who have different roles and different health plans that change annually. This should give an idea about the waste of time and resources encountered on a daily basis.

Johns Hopkins health system deals with about 700 different health plans. The complexity this creates led to its own redundancies in several departments in their health system and was calculated to be more than $40 million annually [5].

Health systems have what we call prior authorization departments and their job is to work on approving interventions from insurance companies. This is not only demanding in means of man power and cost but in many instances can delay patient care as the paper work process for approval can take a long time.

57

If a conflict between the ordering provider and insurance company exists, then an appeal process can be started in which the physician will write an appeal letter citing most recent literature and justification for the requested intervention. The insurance company may or may not accept the appeal (in my experience, they almost never accept it) and the next step will be a peer to peer discussion, where the physician and an insurance company physician consultant will talk over the phone to discuss the case and the need for the intervention (in my experience, this rarely works). This can give you an idea again on how much time and effort is wasted every day across the country. This difficult and laborious process in an attempt to perform routine regular work creates another distraction for the physician on top of all other competing demands.

In addition to the external complexity, each system will have its internal complexity. Each system will have a pyramidal structure that can make it hard for physicians to make their own decisions that can often be related to patient care. A physician will have to go to his / her bosses, sometimes needing to go all the way to the top of the pyramid to get permission, a process that can take several months or more for a simple action/decision.

It is interesting that most of the health care related regulations and policies are written by non-physicians, which further complexifies the process. More regulations will not take into account the reality and needs of a physician as the authors do not see the day to day practice of a physician and patients' needs in the health system.

There are many other regulations that do not have any literature or research backing and lead to a waste of drugs, time, and resources. This in turn leads to a financial burden for health systems, higher cost for insurance companies and patients.

The sustainability of these practices may not be achievable due to the associated high cost. The cost per capita per year for healthcare in the US is almost twice the cost in other comparable advanced countries. However surprisingly, health outcomes were not any better than those countries and were actually worse in some cases. So, the US has more spending but equal or worse results [6].

58

References

1. The bureaucratic hassles physicians face are extraordinary Peter Ubel. Physician, August 2016.

2. An epidemic of disillusioned doctors https://danielleofri.com/an-epidemic-of-disillusioned-doctors/

3. Bureaucrats are killing private medical practice by Mark Howshar, 2014.

4. Field RI. Why is health care regulation so complex?. P T. 2008; 33(10):607-8.

5. Is Insurance Bureaucracy Lengthening Physician Workdays? https://healthcare.dmagazine.com/2014/07/21/is-insurance-bureaucracy-lengthening-physician-workdays/

6. Papanicolas I, Woskie LR, Jha AK. Health Care Spending in the United States and Other High-Income Countries. JAMA. 2018; 319(10):1024–1039.

BURNOUT

Burnout is a problem that can begin even before starting medical school. Students study very hard in undergrad to get into medical school, the competition is very aggressive, and only the best will make it to medical school. The risk for burnout continues during medical school and worsens during residency.

During training a resident may believe that the burnout and agony will conclude with the end of their residency training, but surprisingly this is not the case. Burnout may continue thereafter, until retirement.

Physicians work long hours and depending on the setting, hours may vary. A private practice physician who owns their practice with no other partners will need to be available and on call 24/7. Only if practice grows, will it reduce the hours or frequency of being on call.

Many factors can lead to burnout, ranging from long work hours to dealing with complex patient care situations. 54% of physicians show at least one symptom of burnout. Emergency Department physicians have the highest burnout rates, with 20 % of residents indicating they fell asleep while driving due to fatigue related to work. A large survey showed that about 7 % of physicians consider suicide annually, which is an incredibly alarming statistic.

Seven out of ten physicians mentioned they will never recommend their profession to their kids or family members [1].

Burnout starts when the physician feels emotionally and physically exhausted, working for long hours to the point where it becomes hard to recover during non-work hours. This can lead to a negative attitude towards patients, and lead to the physician being less responsive to patient needs.

Over time the physician may feel a lack of value, and their hopes and dreams fade. Medicine may become a routine job that the physician has to do for daily living. Burnout is the loss of passion.

Some reasons for physician burnout include, but are not limited to:

1. The nature of practicing medicine. Physicians work long hours, dealing with sick and dying people. Not only do they deal with the patient, but they also deal with the patient's family members who also have worries and anxiety related to their loved one's condition. Physicians have to always be available to answer questions for the patient and their family members. Physicians may get called at any time of the day when they are on call. They are called at midnight, 3 am, 4 am, occasionally for simple questions that do not require emergent treatment.

2. The physician does not only deal with patients and clinical care (that would be the dream) but physicians also deal with policies, bureaucracy, and regulations that change from year to year, even from month to month. Physicians also have to deal with their compensation plan which is very inconsistent. Physicians' salaries can change from year to year depending on different variables, so many worry about how much they will be paid the following year.

   Having a life. Students in medical school do not learn about work life balance. As we discussed before, medical school is a competitive and stressful environment that does not account for anything other than competition and achievement. Stresses of regular life, such as an argument with a spouse, having a sick child, school meetings, taking kids to their activities, finances and more can also lead to poor work-life balance [2].

3. Medical students graduate with characteristics that make them workaholics, perfectionists, a misconceived superhero, and may be pessimistic. Physicians put patients first, but frequently forget that if they are burned out, they will not be able to provide the best care for their patients.

4. Having a bad boss. If the boss does not have good leadership skills, this is really tough. So, in addition to all those stressors, having a leader that will not support you is another huge stressor. People do not quit their jobs but quit their boss. One study demonstrated that there is a strong direct relationship between the quality of the boss and job satisfaction and burnout [3]. It is common in the medical field that with the change in leadership, several physicians will leave

the workplace because they simply cannot get along with the new boss.

Burned out physicians may suffer from poor memory, lack of attention, and poor decision making which can lead to poor patient care, complications, inappropriate patient management, and heavier cost on the health system.

There is a strong relationship between burnout and the incidence of major medical errors [4-5]. In fact, studies showed that emotional exhaustion among physicians predict a higher mortality rate among their patients [6].

Burnout also leads to decreased patient satisfaction, possibly related to poor communication with patients [7-8].

Unfortunately, if a physician is burned out it can lead to poor interpersonal interactions, impact patient satisfaction, and result in poor scores on patient satisfaction surveys. The results of these surveys can used when determining the physician's salary, and if the complaints are too abundant, the physician may undergo disciplinary action or even lose their job.

Although the majority of physicians are caring and provide excellent care, burnout can have a negative impact on the ability of a good physician to provide the highest quality care. Only if we address the issue of burnout among physicians can we create an environment where physicians are supported, and therefore can provide the highest level of care to their patients.

References

1. The physician burnout crisis. https://www.lightning-bolt.com/physician-burnout crisis/?gclid=Cj0KCQiAnNXiBRCoARIsAJe_1cp6wvnmHcf62T wsSVasedz7AJiXnVj9wzg_DubdU65q7vDNxrD7yoaAm2XEAL w_wcB

2. Dyrbye LN, Sotile W, Boone S, et al. A survey of U.S. physicians and their partners regarding the impact of work-home conflict. *J Gen Intern Med.* 2014; 29(1):155–161.

3. Shanafelt T, Gorringe G, Menaker R, et al. Impact of organizational leadership on physician burnout and satisfaction. Mayo Clin Proc. 2015; 90(4):432–440.

4. Hayashino Y, UtsugiOzaki M , Feldman M , et al . Hope modified the association between distress and incidence of self-perceived medical errors among practicing physicians: prospective cohort study. PLoS One 2012;7: e35585

5. Shanafelt TD , Balch CM , Bechamps G , et al. Burnout and medical errors among American surgeons. Ann Surg 2010; 251:995–1000

6. Dewa CS, Loong D, Bonato S, Trojanowski L. The relationship between physician burnout and quality of healthcare in terms of safety and acceptability: a systematic review. BMJ Open. 2017 Jun 21;7(6): e015141.

7. Ratanawongsa N, Roter D, Beach MC, et al. Physician burnout and patient-physician communication during primary care encounters. J Gen Intern Med 2008; 23:1581–8

8. Travado L, Grassi L, Gil F, et al. Physician-patient communication among Southern European cancer physicians: the influence of psychosocial orientation and burnout. Psychooncology 2005; 14:661–70

ARE PHYSICIANS WELL VALUED?

The health system has undergone significant changes in the past decade, including modification of the health system structure and payment models. Many physicians felt excluded from this process, which directly impacted them.

A survey of 980 US physicians in 8 specialties demonstrated that physicians did not feel sufficiently engaged in making important decisions about cost control, performance improvement, and adoption of new reimbursement models. In addition, physicians felt overruled by hospitals and managers without having the opportunity to provide sufficient input.

It has been well proven that physicians who do not participate in decision-making tend to be more resistant to their systems as compared to physicians who participate in the decision-making process [1].

Junior physicians in the UK reported they do not feel valued, although they work hard for long hours. This is likely the same case in the US [2].

A recent survey by the Royal College of Physicians showed some interesting results. Researchers found that more than 50% of the time, 78% of consultants felt valued by patients and 70% by colleagues and staff but surprisingly, only 26 % felt being valued by the hospital they work for [3].

A contributing factor to physician dissatisfaction is not feeling valued, and that the majority of medical policies and plans are decided and implemented by lawmakers, administrators, insurance companies and others. While I have to admit that in some instances, decision makers will consult with physicians, this is not always the case.

Excluding physicians from decision making is not ideal, and if providers do not feel valued, this may impact their career, satisfaction, and patient care.

I witnessed several physicians who left their work place for not feeling valued, and unfortunately this is a common occurrence. Physicians work long hours and dedicate a lot for their livelihood to build their career; so not feeling valued can hit them hard. I have also witnessed physicians who will completely quit practicing medicine because they do not feel valued.

References

1. Doctors Feel Excluded from Health Care Value Efforts https://hbr.org/2017/10/doctors-feel-excluded-from-health-care-value-efforts

2. Significant work still do to make junior doctors feel valued http://www.nationalhealthexecutive.com/Health-Care-News/hee-significant-work-still-do-to-make-junior-doctors-feel-valued

3. Wellbeing survey finds majority of consultants do not feel valued by their hospital. https://www.rcplondon.ac.uk/news/wellbeing-survey-finds-majority-consultants-do-not-feel-valued-their-hospital

ERRORS IN THE MEDICAL FIELD

Physicians, including those in training, are not allowed to make errors. Errors happen in all professions; however, the stakes are often very high for physicians. A single error may cause disability or death, and irrevocably change many lives forever.

Physicians are human, and therefore will occasionally make mistakes. Fortunately, most errors are minor and do not results in adverse outcomes to the patient. Errors due to negligence or those that lead to serious adverse outcomes are not common. and have to be addressed very seriously. Unfortunately, minor errors are occasionally taken to an extreme level and can risk a physician's career.

This is one of the hardest and most important topics to discuss. Physicians work hard, for long hours, are commonly sleep deprived, and face many challenges. This creates a culture that easily facilitates errors.

Burnout has been identified as a main reason for physician errors. A large survey performed indicated that physicians suffering burnout report twice as many errors as physicians who do not suffer burnout [1].

Several studies indicate that most medical errors are related to system flaws [2-5]. The Institute of Medicine indicated that out of 98,000 reported hospital deaths attributed to medical errors each year, 90% are the result of failed systems and procedures [2]. Putting systems and structures in place will minimize the risk for errors, however, it does not address the larger problem of physician burnout.

References

1. Physicians burnout is a big factor in medical errors. https://www.futurity.org/medical-errors-physician-burnout-1811152/

2. Kohn LT, Corrigan JM, Donaldson MS (eds): To err is human: Building a safer health system. Washington, DC, National Academies Press, 2000

3. Rason J. Human error. Cambridge, England: Cambridge University Press; 1990.

4. Leape L. Error in medicine. JAMA. 1994; 272:1851-7.

5. Bogner MS (ed). Human error in Medicine. Hillsdale, NJ: Lawrence Erl-baum Associates, 1994.

PHYSICIANS AND ADDICTION

It is estimated that 10-12% of physicians will develop a substance abuse disorder during their career, which is higher than the general population [1-2].

There is a social stigma that physicians with addictions face, which may lead to them not seeking help. Without help addition can eventually lead to mortality, due to overdose or suicide [3]. In addition, an addicted physician can put patient care in jeopardy and place their livelihood at risk.

A cohort conducted over a 5-year period included 904 physicians, 87 % of them were enrolled in state physician health programs, 50.3 % indicated that alcohol was the highest abused substance, 35.9 % for opioids, 7.9 % for stimulants in and 5.9 % marked other substances represented. 50 % indicated they abused more than one substance. 17 % indicated previous treatment for addiction.

Some specialties are known to have higher incidence including Anesthesiology, Emergency Medicine, and Psychiatry.

It is important to notice that physicians have easy access to medications, which makes them exposed on a daily basis to these drugs. If a physician feels down for even a short duration of time, he/she may decide to try using these drugs which are very handy and then it is a slippery slope from there. Now the important question is, shall we allow addicted physicians to re-enter practice after recovery?

Physicians tend to have a high abstinence rate after recovery from addiction, even higher than the general population. The abstinence rate is estimated to be 74-90 % in physicians after recovery [4-5].

Other reports showed that 25 % of recovering physicians will have at least 1 relapse [6].

Risk of relapse increased by family history of substance abuse and the presence of a psychiatric illness. While the incidence of relapse may seem to be low, it can be fatal, 16 % of relapsed anesthesia residents were found dead before a relapse was suspected.

When a physician is found to be having a substance abuse disorder, the hospital will remove this physician from any patient care responsibilities, the issue will be reported to the state medical board. They will then go into a rehab program and request to practice again after a formal recovery.

Requests have to be approved at the state level first which is not guaranteed. If approved, this physician will then apply for jobs again and hospitals may or may not accept the physician to work for concern of relapse and patient care issues. Sometimes the ideal situation is the physician apply for certain positions that guarantee he/she will not have access to addictive medications. Sometimes there is no way back to practice and this is simply the end of their career. It is a long, complex, and agonizing process with an unknown outcome. Again, any serious error a physician makes can simply terminate his/her career forever.

The physician may find him/herself one day with no income, still needing to pay all accumulated loans in addition to daily living expenses, a very tough situation.

Addiction in a physician can be suspected if he/she is requesting night shifts, using addictive drugs more than others, falling asleep at the work place, volunteering to give lunch breaks in the operating rooms, smell of alcohol, narrow pupils, repeated errors in paper work, requesting too frequent bathroom breaks, and the presence of financial and/or family stresses.

While a physician may pursue addiction due to burnout and other work-related stresses discussed in this book, addiction must be addressed and dealt with as it compromises quality of patient care.

References

1. Hughes PH, Brandenburg N, Baldwin DC Jr, et al. Prevalence of substance use among US physicians JAMA. 1992;267(17):2333-2339.

2. McLellan AT, Skipper GS, Campbell M, DuPont RL. Five-year outcomes in a cohort study of physicians treated for substance use disorders in the United States. BMJ. 2008; 337:a2038.

3. Myers MF, Gabbard GO. The Physician as Patient: A Clinical Handbook for Mental Health Professionals. Washington, DC: American Psychiatric Publishing; 2008.

4. Skutar C. Physicians Recovery Network targets attitudes about impairment. Mich Med. 1990;89(12):30-32.

5. Kliner DJ, Spicer J, Barnett P. Treatment outcome of alcoholic physicians. J Stud Alcohol. 1980;41(11):1217-1220.

6. Domino KB, Hornbein TF, Polissar NL, et al. Risk factors for relapse in health care professionals with substance use disorders. JAMA. 2005;293(12): 1453-1460.

7. Menk EJ, Baumgarten RK, Kingsley CP, Culling RD, Middaugh R. Success of reentry into anesthesiology training programs by residents with a history of substance abuse. JAMA. 1990;263(22):3060-3062.

PHYSICIANS AND SUICIDE

I will be discussing, in this chapter, one of the most difficult topics. I have personally felt the pain of colleagues and friends, who are physicians, commit suicide. We always hear about this before entering our training but when it actually happens, I cannot describe to you how painful it is. Hearing that one of my colleagues committed suicide is one of the most painful things that has ever happened to me. The first questions that came to my mind are, "Did I miss anything?" "Were there signs that I could have paid attention to?" "Could I have done anything to avoid this tragedy?"

This sad painful feeling can be associated with a sense of guilt especially if we look back and find that our colleague actually was experiencing stressors that we should have reported.

The death of a beloved one is painful in itself but when it is suicide, it hits much differently.

The issue of physicians' suicide has been reported since 1858, over 150 years ago. The problem continues to this day and the numbers are increasing.

The statistics regarding suicide among physicians is quite frightening. Literature reported that suicide among physicians are 2-3 times higher than the general population. This is estimated to be the equivalent of 2 entire medical school classes committing suicide a year.
While the number is already high, some literature indicated that this number is even underestimated as sometimes the cause of death is labelled as accidental or an unplanned overdose, or any other cause.

It has been reported that physicians that harm themselves can potentially be of harm to their patients and families.

I personally read several cases where the physician killed his spouse and then committed suicide. If you look online, you will find many of these cases. Although a physician can be extremely successful, social problems encountered can make a physician's perception skewed [1-2].

In 2018, it was estimated that one physician commits suicide in the US every day. It has been confirmed that this is the highest rate of suicide among all professions, estimated to total 28 – 40 per 100,000 physicians [3].

It has been proposed that physicians who commit suicide are likely depressed or suffer other psychiatric problems.

It was also surprising for me to know that the suicide rate among physicians is higher than that among the military which is a very stressful job. I have cared for many of our veterans who suffered extreme stresses during their time in the military service especially ones previously deployed to a war zone region.

Studies also showed that female physicians attempt suicide much less often than women in other professions, but their completion rate exceeded that of the general population by 2.5-4 times [3].

Suicide among physicians can be related to mood disorders, alcoholism, and /or substance abuse.

Depression prevalence among physicians is 12% for male physicians, and 9.5 % for female physicians. Rates are higher in medical students and residents.

Some physicians will have symptoms and signs of depression and other mood disorders, but they tend not to seek medical care due to the stigma around being seen by a psychiatrist and being labelled as mentally ill.

I always wondered if a physician is diagnosed with a mood disorder or depression, will this risk their career? Will their hospital allow them to practice? Maybe these are fears that all physicians have and cause them not to seek help.

Literature also reports that physicians who commit suicide may look very happy on the outside, but the problem runs deep down and remains in silence.

Poisoning and hanging seem to be the most common two methods used by physicians to commit suicide. Physicians also have access to many drugs that when used in high doses can be lethal [3].

A significant number of physicians commit suicide in the hospital and have been found dead in the call room. They tend to overdose in the hospital, hang themselves, and sometimes shoot themselves.

Training during medical school, residency, and fellowship is mostly about survival, being strong, and staying away from trouble. The high pressure, stress and competition makes the graduate set different standards.

Failing medical board exams and unlatching for residency have been identified as reasons for suicide.

Another important figure: 23 % of interns (first year residents) have suicidal thoughts; this amounts to 1 in 4 interns [4].

Internship specifically is very stressful as it is the first year after medical school, the first year a medical student will become a physician, experience the long hours and care for very sick patients while they are not very knowledgeable due to little experience. While interns should have enough support from their senior residents and faculty, sometimes the high workload make this difficult.

Students dream of being rich, living in a big mansion, having a beautiful family, but all of the sudden the dream can change once they enter medical school. They find themselves in all the stress I have described, in a competitive and cutthroat environment. Many students do not recognize the amount of effort and time they need to put into medical school to be able to succeed.

While it may seem surprising, it was found that family members of physicians who commit suicide are themselves at higher risk for committing suicide and they tend to commit suicide in the same way.

An average physician in the USA will care for about 2,300 patients. It is estimated that 1 million patients will lose their caring physician every year.

A small percent of physicians who commit suicide will also commit homicide and usually the homicide will include killing the partner or spouse.

During my medical school and training I have seen several colleagues who leave medical school or quit residency because they were not successful. All I can say is they did the right thing. Changing their career at any point is much better than failing, committing suicide, or living forever an unhappy life with the inability to cope with the job requirements.

References

1. RELATIONSHIPS; THE STRESS IN DOCTORS' FAMILIES - The New York Times 10/21/18, 2(14 PM https://www.nytimes.com/1982/03/08/style/relationships-the-stress-in-doctors-families.html Page 2 of 3

2. Wible P. What I've learned from my tally of 757 doctor suicides. Ideal Medical Care website. idealmedicalcare.org/blog/ive-learned-547-doctor-suicides. Published October 28, 2017. Accessed January 28, 2018.

3. American Psychiatric Association 2018 annual meeting, May 5, 2018. Deepika Tanwar, MD, psychiatric program, Harlem Hospital Center, New York. Beth Brodsky, PhD, associate clinical professor of medical psychology in psychiatry, Columbia University and Irving Medical Center, New York.

4. Guille, C., Zhao, Z., Krystal, J., Nichols, B., Brady, K., & Sen, S. (2015). Web-Based Cognitive Behavioral Therapy Intervention for the Prevention of Suicidal Ideation in Medical Interns. JAMA Psychiatry, 72(12), 1192.

QUITTING MEDICINE

Due to the multiple stressors physicians suffer, many physicians are leaving medicine mid-career. Others are decreasing their working hours and days or moving towards part-time appointments.

These changes are concerning as this may lead to decrease in the number of providers who provide medical care. It is estimated that by 2030, our country will have and estimated physician's shortage of 100,000 according to a study commissioned by the American Association of Medical Colleges [1].

Quitting medicine is a problem we have to work on so that our nation does not find itself in a difficult situation in the future. It is not only about a physician shortage, but I foresee that working physicians will have a much higher burnout due to the increased demand and the need to keep up with care.

There are several surveys that confirm this fact. Another national survey indicated that due to the low compensation and hassles of health care reform, 34 % of physicians are planning on quitting Medicine in the next decade [1].

Another online survey that included 2,218 physicians indicated that 16 % of respondents are strongly considering retirement, leaving medicine or shifting to part time in 2012. Physicians who participated in this survey provided lengthy and emotional responses which indicates their situation and the culture they work in. Physicians in certain specialties reported that more than 50 % will retire in the next 10 years [1].

Another comprehensive survey that included 13, 575 US physicians indicated challenges in patient access and a significant growing concern of physicians' shortage [1]. It was found that physicians are moving towards working fewer hours, seeing fewer patients and trying to limit the access to their practices due to the regulations that mandates physicians an enormous amount of paper work and admin duties related to patient care.

It is estimated that if no appropriate solutions are put in place soon for this problem, 44,250 full time equivalent physicians will be lost from the workforce in the next 4 years.

81

100,000 physicians are planning to move from practice owners to be employees of health systems, leading to 91 million less patient encounters, which in turn will reflect on access and patient care [1].

In 2016, about 60 % of medical school graduates from Stanford said they plan to go into business, research or consulting rather than direct patient care [2].

Leaving medicine is a problem in other countries as well. 4 in 10 United Kingdom (UK) medical students indicated that they or someone they know has considered quitting medicine due to financial stresses.

In addition, one survey showed that 100 medical students in the UK have quit over the past 5 years. Financial and mental health pressures were the key factors to blame [3].

Another survey of 100 students found 60% of them experienced financial stressors with 65 % of this subgroup also mentioning its impact on their mental health and well-being [4].

Sometimes the answer is not completely quitting medicine but quitting patient care. Several physicians are moving to medical administrative jobs either in universities, health systems, or pharmaceutical companies. Some see this as an opportunity to continue to be in the medical field without facing the stresses of patient care directly.

I am not saying that all physician leaders did it for this purpose; very good physician leaders are needed in non-patient care areas to indirectly enhance patient care.

If you look online for physicians' jobs, you will find countless positions in all specialties in all states. While this might be perceived as a good job market for physicians, this also means we have a massive shortage and if we do not find a solution, it will only get worse.

There has been a movement of establishing groups on Facebook and other social media platforms for physicians to consult each other about quitting medicine. The numbers of physicians who join those groups are in thousands.

If you look online, you will find many heart-breaking stories about physicians who after going to medical school, residency training, and sometimes fellowship training, quit medicine. Having finally achieved their life dream by becoming a physician, are suddenly faced with the reality of burnout, long hours of work, bureaucracy, and low salaries. Each physician wrote his/her story very emotionally, as giving up on a life dream is not easy.

Some physicians when telling their stories indicated that many physicians will do the job because they need the paycheck and because they have no other skills that will allow them to pursue another career. In addition, they have children and medical school loans to pay, so no other options.

Several described that they found support in the online groups and talking to a career coach which guided them to finally make the decision of quitting medicine after having an alternative career planned and some end up quitting without a plan.

References

1. A Survey of America's Physicians: Practice Patterns and Perspectives https://physiciansfoundation.org/focus-areas/a-survey-of-americas-physicians-practice-patterns-and-perspectives/

2. Mamas, Don't Let Your Babies Grow Up To Be Doctors https://www.forbes.com/sites/realspin/2017/01/06/mamas-dont-let-your-babies-grow-up-to-be-doctors/#1590717c4199

3. Medical schools lose 200 students a year amid money and mental health pressure https://www.gponline.com/medical-schools-lose-200-students-year-amid-money-mental-health-pressure/article/1519116

4. Nunez-Mulder L. Medical students consider abandoning degree because of financial pressures, survey finds. BMJ. 2018 Nov 26; 363:k4990.

DIVERSITY AS AN ADDITIVE STRESSOR FOR PHYSICIANS

Diversity is becoming a serious issue in the medical filed. Diversity can be represented by sex, gender, religion, color, ethnicity, country of origin, being a foreign medical graduate, and more. Physicians belonging to minority groups have reported discrimination at all phases in their career. This is another big stressor in addition to the stressors I have discussed. It is very important to ensure equity and fairness among all physicians at all levels without discrimination.

I want each reader to think of how it feels if you hide your identity every day for many years for the fear of discrimination. Even worse, think of if you disclose it and then receive discrimination in a very intense and stressful culture.

It has been reported that only 2.7% of medical students report disability while it is believed that the number is much higher. There is fear that disclosing disability may impact their future career.

I will be briefly discussing the most important diversities in the medical field in the next few short chapters.

WOMEN PHYSICIANS

Women represent only one third of physicians in the US and mostly in areas such as family medicine, obstetrics, gynecology and pediatrics.

Based on data from the Association of American Medical College (AAMC) only 15 % of department chairs are women and only 16 % are deans. By 2012, only 18 % of CEOs were women [1].

Several studies have documented the presence of gender differences in achievements and compensation in medicine. Other studies also documented the presence of gender differences in faculty ranking among physicians [2-11].

Several surveys indicated that women are paid significantly less than men in the medical field after adjusting for specialty, work hours, years of experience, and family structure. The same finding was reported in academic medicine.

Although it is important to point to the weakness of these studies and the presence of many limitations [12-21].

I have read online about female physicians, while in their training, that would try to hide their pregnancy for the fear of losing an opportunity or not being able to get a job immediately. It has been reported that male residents may not be happy about this, as female residents may need to take a maternity leave, which will further increase their work hours and duty coverage during their colleagues leave of absence.

Covering is a behavior that is sought by a person to reduce the stigma by reducing obtrusiveness of an identity.

One report performed in 2013 indicated that 61 % (of 3,129 professionals), reported covering one or more identity [22].

Discrimination against women in the medical field has been reported in other countries across the world as well.

References

1. Sexism Is Alive, Well in the Healthcare Industry https://www.healthline.com/health-news/sexism-is-alive-in-healthcare#1

2. Jolliff L, Leadley J, Coakley E, Sloane RA. Women in US academic medicine and science: statistics and benchmarking report, 2011–2012. https://www.aamc.org/download/415556/data/2011-2012wimsstatsreport.pdf. Published 2012. Accessed June 9, 2016.

3. Nickerson KG, Bennett NM, Estes D, Shea S. The status of women at one academic medical center: breaking through the glass ceiling. *JAMA*. 1990;264(14):1813-1817.

4. Kaplan SH, Sullivan LM, Dukes KA, Phillips CF, Kelch RP, Schaller JG. Sex differences in academic advancement: results of a national study of pediatricians. *N Engl J Med*. 1996;335(17):1282-1289.PubMedGoogle ScholarCrossref

5. Nonnemaker L. Women physicians in academic medicine: new insights from cohort studies. *N Engl J Med*. 2000;342(6):399-405.

6. Tesch BJ, Wood HM, Helwig AL, Nattinger AB. Promotion of women physicians in academic medicine: glass ceiling or sticky floor? *JAMA*. 1995;273(13):1022-1025.

7. Wallis LA, Gilder H, Thaler H. Advancement of men and women in medical academia: a pilot study. *JAMA*. 1981;246(20):2350-2353.

8. Carr PL, Friedman RH, Moskowitz MA, Kazis LE. Comparing the status of women and men in academic medicine. *Ann Intern Med*. 1993;119(9):908-913.

9. Eloy JA, Svider PF, Cherla DV, et al. Gender disparities in research productivity among 9952 academic physicians. *Laryngoscope*. 2013;123(8):1865-1875.

10. Reed DA, Enders F, Lindor R, McClees M, Lindor KD. Gender differences in academic productivity and leadership appointments of physicians throughout academic careers. *Acad Med.* 2011;86(1):43-47.

11. Jena AB, Khullar D, Ho O, Olenski AR, Blumenthal DM. Sex differences in academic rank in US medical schools in 2014. *JAMA.* 2015;314(11):1149-1158.

12. Baker LC. Differences in earnings between male and female physicians. *N Engl J Med.* 1996;334(15):960-964.

13. Lo Sasso AT, Richards MR, Chou CF, Gerber SE. The $16,819 pay gap for newly trained physicians: the unexplained trend of men earning more than women. *Health Aff (Millwood).* 2011;30(2):193-201.

14. Seabury SA, Chandra A, Jena AB. Trends in the earnings of male and female health care professionals in the United States, 1987 to 2010. *JAMA Intern Med.* 2013;173(18):1748-1750.

15. Hoff TJ. Doing the same and earning less: male and female physicians in a new medical specialty. *Inquiry.* 2004;41(3):301-315.

16. Jagsi R, Griffith KA, Stewart A, Sambuco D, DeCastro R, Ubel PA. Gender differences in the salaries of physician researchers. *JAMA.* 2012;307(22):2410-2417.

17. Jagsi R, Griffith KA, Stewart A, Sambuco D, DeCastro R, Ubel PA. Gender differences in salary in a recent cohort of early-career physician-researchers. *Acad Med.* 2013;88(11):1689-1699.

18. Ash AS, Carr PL, Goldstein R, Friedman RH. Compensation and advancement of women in academic medicine: is there equity? *Ann Intern Med.* 2004;141(3):205-212.

19. Weeks WB, Wallace TA, Wallace AE. How do race and sex affect the earnings of primary care physicians? *Health Aff (Millwood).* 2009;28(2):557-566.

20. Ness RB, Ukoli F, Hunt S, et al. Salary equity among male and female internists in Pennsylvania. *Ann Intern Med.* 2000;133(2):104-110.
21. DesRoches CM, Zinner DE, Rao SR, Iezzoni LI, Campbell EG. Activities, productivity, and compensation of men and women in the life sciences. *Acad Med.* 2010;85(4):631-639.

22. Diversity and Inclusion in Medical Schools: The Reality https://blogs.scientificamerican.com/voices/diversity-and-inclusion-in-medical-schools-the-reality/

Foreign medical graduates (FMGs)

Foreign Medical Graduates (FMGs) represent a considerable portion of physicians practicing in the US. Based on published data, we will need more FMGs to fill the huge deficit we will have in the next decade. FMGs already been filling the gap for a long time for the reasons we mentioned in previous parts of this book.

One thing I noticed when I applied for residency in the US was that there are websites that will advise on what is called FMG friendly and non-friendly programs. So, it is clear here that some programs welcome FMGs and some do not.

One article actually stated that USA owes a huge dept of gratitude to non-US trained physicians [1].

I think the reason for this gratitude is FMGs have always filled the gaps to provide good health care in the US as the number of US graduates is not sufficient to provide coverage to the entire country.

I am also aware that other countries now have a deficit in numbers of physicians due to the move of physicians to Western countries. It is a fact that several countries are suffering the decrease in number of physicians for multiple reasons.

Although FMGs played an important role in the health system in the USA, some educators seem to be embarrassed when they mentioned they have FMGs in their programs [2].
Foreign-born physicians reported that they face more insensitivity, discrimination, and isolation at the workplace.

In Sweden, foreign born physicians face higher levels of threats and violence from patients as compared to native physicians in addition to reporting harassment from their colleagues.

In Germany, they reported discrimination in the workplace [3-6].

Literature showed that US programs discriminated against FMGs during the residency application process.

A survey of directors of surgical residency programs showed that 70 % of them indicated that FMGs were discriminated against in the residency application process.

27 % of physicians indicated that patients and their relatives were the main source of discrimination, while it was 10 % from superiors and management and 12 % from colleagues and coworkers [7].

Discrimination against FMGs was not limited to the residency applications process but also has been reported in barriers of obtaining licensure, limited practice options, and lack of acceptance from peers [8].

In the early 1990s, proposals were submitted to congress to decrease the number of physicians in training programs to 100% the number of American graduates, the purpose of this was suggested to decrease the number of FMGs who will be able to join training programs.

Some proposed that FMGs may perform lower quality work than US graduates but based on literature this was proven to be incorrect, the quality of care provided by US and non-US
medical graduates did not show any significant difference [9].

Another finding that was extremely interesting was that the proportion of FMGs in a residency program was found to be significantly and inversely related to the program desirability. So, programs with large numbers of FMGs will not be as desirable for US applicants [10-11].

Reports showed that immigrant physicians are subject to discrimination and bullying from their colleagues. Commonly they will show it as talking down to them due to their accent, or the way they dress especially for certain physicians who come from countries where they have different traditional clothing, hair covers, and the way they deal with their names that can be difficult to say sometimes.

Immigrant physicians also reported discrimination and harassment from administrators. Physicians mentioned they were told things like, "this is not how we do it here". In addition, they get more frequent poor peer reviews and get harsher evaluation compared to their non-minority colleagues.

94

They also reported discrimination and harassment from patients who will treat them differently, and that may have a lack of trust in their abilities or for no obvious reason other than racism [12].

References

1. Gastel B. Impact of International Medical Graduates on U.S. and Global Health Care: summary of the ECFMG 50th anniversary invitational conference. Acad Med. 2006 Dec;81(12 Suppl):S3-6.

2. Centor R: What I Have Learned from IMGs. SGIM Forum 2007, 30:3-12

3. Chen PG, Curry LA, Bernheim SM, Berg D, Gozu A, Nunez-Smith M. Professional challenges of non-U.S.-born international medical graduates and recommendations for support during residency training. Acad Med. 2011;86(11):1383–1388.

4. Eneroth M, Gustafsson Senden M, Schenck Gustafsson K, Wall M, Fridner A. Threats or violence from patients was associated with turnover intention among foreign-born GPs - a comparison of four workplace factors associated with attitudes of wanting to quit one's job as a GP. Scand J Prim Health Care. 2017;35(2):208–213.

5. Wall M, Schenck-Gustafsson K, Gustafsson Senden M, Eneroth M, Fridner A. Work environment and harassment among primary care physicians. In: International Conference of Physician Health: 2014. *London, England*; 2014.

6. Klingler C, Marckmann G. Difficulties experienced by migrant physicians working in German hospitals: a qualitative interview study. Hum Resour Health. 2016;14(1):57.

7. Desbiens NA, Vidaillet HJ Jr. Discrimination against international medical graduates in the United States residency program selection process. BMC Med Educ. 2010 Jan 25; 10:5.

8. Haveliwala YA. Problems of foreign-born psy- chiatrists. Psychiatr Q. 1979; 51:307-311.

9. Mick SS, Comfort ME. The quality of care of international medical graduates: how does it com- pare to that of US medical graduates? Med Care Res Rev. 1997; 54:379-413.

10. Riley JD, Hannis M, Rice KG. Are international medical graduates a factor in residency program selection? A survey of fourth-year medical stu- dents. Acad Med.1996; 71:381-386.

11. Whitcomb ME, Miller RS. Comparison of IMG- dependent and non-IMG-dependent residencies in the national Resident Matching Program. JAMA 1996; 276:700-703.

12. Doctors Face Racism in Medicine https://www.mdmag.com/physicians-money-digest/contributor/heidi-moawad-md/2016/11/doctors-face-racism-in-medicine

PHYSICIANS OF COLOR

A letter written by Frederick Irving in 1942 to the Dean of Harvard Medical School detailed his embarrassment and discomfort over the admission of 2 colored medical students. He further recommended in his letter that the students should be withdrawn if any questions or concerns are raised by patients. Reading about this in the year 2018 may sound trivial, but the lack of acceptance of diversity still exists. While it may not be written and documented about it is noticed in people's behaviors [1].

One report evaluated 155 medical schools from 1908 to 1910. During that time, 7 black medical schools were in operation. Based on the recommendations of the reporter, 2 schools were closed and during that time African-Americans were denied admittance into white medical institutions.

The reporter also adopted new standards for admission to medical schools that made it very difficult for African-Americans to go to medical school. And they were not able to be enrolled in all US medical schools until 1966.

Between the 1950s and 1960s, African-Americans made up 10 % of the total population but only 2.2 % of US physicians.

The number of African-Americans, Hispanics, and Native Americans increased to be more than one third of the US population in 2008 but represented only 8.7% of physicians [2].

I have to admit that there has been a lot of good work to increase the numbers and make it a fair process, but it seems there is still an under-representation for African-American physicians. Some currently practicing African-American physicians had their education decades ago when discrimination was obvious and apparent.

There have been reports on patients requesting white physicians to avoid seeing African-American physicians. While this might seem unusual for some readers, it actually happens.

References

1. Diversity and Inclusion in Medical Schools: The Reality https://blogs.scientificamerican.com/voices/diversity-and-inclusion-in-medical-schools-the-reality/

2. Report: Too Few Minority Doctors After Decades of Discrimination http://www.cfah.org/hbns/2010/report-too-few-minority-doctors-after-decades-of-discrimination

LGBTQ PHYSICIANS

A report published in academic medicine indicated that 30% of LGBTQ students reported concealing their identity, 40% of them do so from fear of discrimination [1].

Teaching about the LGBTQ population in medical schools is very important. Currently, there is a gap in the current education curriculum.

One study showed that among 427 LGBT physicians 10% reported denial of referrals by their heterosexual colleagues, 15% reported harassment by colleagues, 22% had been socially ostracized, 65% reported hearing a derogatory comment about LGBT individuals, 34% witnessed discrimination in care for an LGBT patient, and 27% witnessed discrimination in treatment of a colleague from the same population [2].

That is why kids, students, medical students, and physicians need training and education on accepting others, no matter what their differences are. People need to understand and accept diversity.

While there is a lot of work and education on certain minority groups, the topic is still much larger and needs to be broader. I do not think anyone can summarize and make a list of all diversity groups. While efforts to improve the situation of certain groups are excellent, the concept of acceptance overall is really what we need.

People need to keep their beliefs to themselves and learn to love all without discrimination.

Nothing is more precious than the human being. We should teach and practice fairness, equity, and acceptance to all.

References

1. Diversity and Inclusion in Medical Schools: The Reality https://blogs.scientificamerican.com/voices/diversity-and-inclusion-in-medical-schools-the-reality/

2. Eliason MJ, Dibble SL, Robertson PA. Lesbian, gay, bisexual, and transgender (LGBT) physicians' experiences in the workplace. J Homosex. 2011;58(10):1355-71.

WOULD YOU RECOMMEND MEDICAL SCHOOL FOR YOUR KIDS?

This is a very important question, are you going to recommend medicine for your kids?

In a survey performed in 2012 including 5,000 physicians 9 out of 10 indicated they will not recommend medicine to their kids [1].

It is noticeable that the most recent generations of medical students are choosing specialties with limited hours, no emergency call and best if they pay well. Honestly, they may have got it right: this will help them to achieve the life work balance assuming they are very passionate and confident they want to become physicians.

While this is good for physicians, what about the patient and who will take care of them if they get sick?

Several of my colleagues advised their children who are interested in the medical filed to pursue a career as a nurse practitioner (NP) or physician assistant (PA). This requires 2-3 years of study, less rigorous than medicine and starting salaries between $85,000 USD and $120,000 USD and more. This is a much higher salary than their colleagues who will be in medical school or residency at that time.

It is estimated that a physician will break even with a NP or PA in the income they make at the age of late 40s given the fact and NP or PA will be working and making income for several years before their class mates who elected to do medicine graduate their training.

I think when we compare the highest pay for an NP or a PA with the lowest pay in medical specialties, I wonder even if they will break even at late 40s, maybe even later in life.

NPs and PAs will typically have a more controlled schedule with certain hours to work on a daily basis and they can elect no work on weekends. I think this is a great work life balance [2].

In my opinion, no one should push his/her kids to go to medical school, this has to be their own choice and after having a full understanding about the career. They have to be passionate about being physicians, accept the struggles that will start on day one, learn that they will compete with the best, they will study for long hours, in addition to understanding what comes after graduation.

References

1. Here's why 9 out of 10 doctors wouldn't recommend medicine as a profession http://america.aljazeera.com/watch/shows/america-tonight/articles/2014/7/9/here-s-why-9 outof10doctorswouldntrecommendmedicineasaprofession.html

2. Mamas, Don't Let Your Babies Grow Up To Be Doctors https://www.forbes.com/sites/realspin/2017/01/06/mamas-dont-let-your-babies-grow-up-to-be-doctors/#1590717c4199

AUTHOR'S MESSAGE

My mom was a physician and she advised me to think very hard before going to medical school. After thinking long and hard about it, and understanding what it takes to become a physician, I decided to follow my passion and go to medical school. My medical school was one of the toughest, if not the toughest in Egypt. I studied for long hours every day, I missed out on social events, hanging out with friends, significant holidays, and family occasions. I was always sleep deprived because I was in extensive competition to remain highly ranked in my class.

In my medical school system, if you rank high in your class, you can be appointed as a faculty at the University. This is an outstanding honor, and an excellent job. So, keeping this in mind, obtaining high rankings was a must for me to continue pursuing my dream of not only being a physician, but being an excellent one. I maintained high ranks throughout my medical school years and I was appointed as a faculty at my medical school.

Then the dream grew, and I wanted to move to the US to learn cutting edge technologies in treating patients. Despite all the challenges facing foreign medical graduates, I did it, and worked very hard to excel at every stage of my training. I prioritized work and school, never caring about how much I slept, the lack of social life, but instead focused on my dream.

I recognized since day one in medical school that this was going to be a long road and will require hard work. I decided I would do whatever it takes to achieve it. I had my ups and downs. But when I reflected on my life, I always knew this is what I wanted, and I kept pursuing it.

Going to medical school has been one of the best decisions I ever made. I go to work happy every day because I know I am helping patients, and nothing is more rewarding than when I am able to cure someone.

The dream is not over, as I still have a lot to achieve in my career. Now that I have more experience, I have learned the importance of keeping my work and home life balanced. I still work hard, and occasionally miss out on important events, but I do a better job being present with my family when I am with them.

I love my career and I believe medicine is a very rewarding job for physicians who do it with passion and love. Looking back, I would still go to medical school and do what I am doing today. Treating patients, saving lives, and improving quality of life by helping patients return to work and enjoy their life with their beloved ones, is worth all of the hard work.

The main point of this book is not to discourage students from going to medical school, but to help them understand what it takes to become a physician so there are no surprises, frustrations, or regrets down the road.

I mentor medical students and when we discuss their future career, it makes me sad that many do not know what it means to be a physician, and the amount of effort they will need to put into their career. Medicine is not for the faint of heart.

I believe that many of the issues we see facing physicians today are due to unrealistic expectations about going to medical school and becoming a doctor. Students believe they will have the most expensive house, a fancy car, a beautiful wife and kids, and be able to vacation in the most desired destinations. While this might be achievable, it will require hard work, long hours, and dealing with many challenges and hardships.

When I was deciding on which fellowship to pursue for my career after my residency training, I talked to my mentor. We discussed the lifestyle and income of each of the different subspecialties. In the end his advice to me was to do what I like to do every day. Income will change with the change of governments, reforms, and even state of work, but being happy going to work every day is the most important factor.

So, the main advice I give to my students, is follow your dreams, be good at what you do, know all what takes to be a physician, and go into the profession with realistic expectations.

Medical students or residents who struggle and end up quitting may feel very frustrated and disappointed that their life dream has just vanished. However, realizing this profession is not for you early is the smartest decision to make, as long as the decision is well thought out. Leaving school and changing your career path early is much better than living miserably after graduation, making errors, or committing suicide later on.

110

It is important in any field to have realistic expectations, goals, and a willingness to do the hard work to achieve those goals. It is important for every person to understand their skills and abilities, so they do not pursue the wrong career path. It is never a bad idea to quit if you cannot do it, just have a detailed plan in mind before you do so to make sure it is not a rash decision made in haste.

I would like also to mention that several physicians live a good life and make very good money but may not have an ideal work-life balance. Many physicians with high incomes work even longer than normal and sacrifice even more. You need to decide if that is worth it for you.

I would like also to stress on the importance of having a mentor. I personally find this a MUST for any person in any career, and especially in medicine. It is difficult to figure out all of this without having a good mentor who can guide the potential physician or applicant to the right path. Mentorship never ends at any point or any phase in the physician's
career. Mentors may change depending on where your career takes you but having someone to help guide you can make a huge difference in your success and happiness.

I find mentorship is needed in all aspects of life, even outside our professional careers. It is better to learn from others' mistakes rather than repeating them yourself.

I truly hope this book will be helpful for the public and aspiring physicians to understand what it takes to be a physician, and for potential physicians to understand the good and bad about being a physician. I also hope it helps patients understand what their physicians go through. The current state of healthcare needs to change so we stop losing physicians to the stress of the job, and instead allow them to return to focusing on being the healer they always dreamed of being.

www.ingramcontent.com/pod-product-compliance
Lightning Source LLC
Chambersburg PA
CBHW072148170526
45158CB00004BA/1551